First published August 2016
Text © Innovations in Pilates, 2016
Published by Innovations in Pilates
with the assistance of Rebus Press
Innovations in Pilates
1 Regina St. Rosanna
VIC 3085 Australia
www.innovationsinpilates.com
Rebus Press
PO Box 622
Hurstbridge VIC 3099
Email: julie@rebuspress.com.au
Web: www.rebuspress.com.au
Anatomy diagrams used with permission of Muscle and Motion
Cover design by Kenyi Diaz
Layout by Kenyi Diaz & Angela Shi
Modelling by Kenyi Diaz, Anthony Lett

National Library of Australia Cataloguing-in-Publication entry

Creator:	Lett, Anthony, author.
Title:	Stretching for Stiffies: A full body Pilates program for people who are stiff in all the wrong places / Anthony Lett, Kenyi Diaz.
ISBN:	978-0-9775099-8-0
Subjects:	Pilates method.
	Health.
	Physical fitness.
Other Creators/ Contributors:	Diaz, Kenyi, author.
Dewey Number:	613.7192

Stretching for Stiffies:

A Full Body Pilates Stretching Program for People Who are Stiff in all the Wrong Places

Anthony Lett / Kenyi Diaz

Anthony

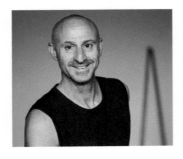

... is a Pilates studio owner, teacher, educator and writer originally from Melbourne Australia. Anthony teaches workshops globally on the material from his books titled *Innovations in Pilates*. Anthony was the Director of Advanced Education for BASI Pilates and has qualifications in philosophy, sports science, exercise medicine and clinical anatomy. Anthony has presented his workshops and keynote addresses in over 25 countries and is a leading creative thinker in the Pilates industry. Anthony's three books contain fascinating world-first 3D Pilates graphics and merge practices from osteopathy, physiotherapy and Yoga with traditional Pilates repertoire. Anthony also created the first *Pilates Anatomy* certification course, as well as the first 3D printed Pilates reformer. *Pilates Anatomy* involves three-dimensional anatomy video, creation of muscles on skeletons, and exploration of functional anatomy in the Pilates studio. Anthony is currently working on a new project titled 'StretchFit'.

anthony@innovationsinpilates.com
http://anthonylett.com.au/
www.innovationsinpilates.com

Kenyi

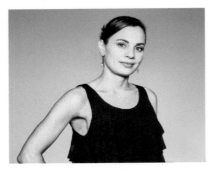

... is a professional Pilates instructor originally from Venezuela, with a background in dance, and training in classical and contemporary Pilates. Kenyi began teaching Pilates in 2004. Kenyi has taught Innovations in Pilates workshops in Australia, Asia, Europe, the UK, South Africa and South America. A skilled graphic artist, Kenyi designed and co-authored all of the *Innovations in Pilates* materials including books, ebooks and video production. Kenyi is pursuing an academic interest in human nutrition; in particular, eating for health and wellbeing, for sports performance, and in the growing area of "food as medicine".

kenyi@innovationsinpilates.com
www.kenyidiaz.com
www.innovationsinpilates.com

Contents

Introduction

This book should be used by teachers or self-practicing students after they have read *Stretching on the Pilates Reformer: Essential Cues and Images*, or *Innovations in Pilates: Therapeutic Muscle Stretching on the Pilates Reformer*. Both books will give you far more detail on the practices recommended including teaching tips, corrections, warm ups, how often to stretch, bony and joint limitations and a whole lot more. In short, they will give you the background depth as a basis to explore the material provided here.

Once you have an underlying understanding of the Innovations in Pilates approach, the next step is to select some material and get to work. Both of the books mentioned discuss the problem of labeling stretching into standards, given that flexibility is joint specific, and that everyone has 'tight bits' and 'looser bits'. In assembling this collection we have selected material for people without much history of stretching, and with less body awareness.

Sometimes, particularly in Yoga, students cannot 'feel' the stretch because they don't know how to organize their body into the correct position in the first place. In this series, we have tried to eliminate that issue. These are stretches that are difficult to get wrong! They target precise regions of the body, and are precise enough to ensure that the body is not able to take the path of least resistance and escape! They also require very little in the way of body awareness or strength to be able to perform.

In essence this collection is simple to cue, biomechanically safe, hard to avoid and effective for anyone who has stiffness in any of the major muscles groups of the body. A few points of discussion before you start...

What if myself or my students don't feel anything?

Sometimes a student will proclaim quite proudly and loudly "I don't feel anything!" My typical response is "Great! This is one small part of your life that does not need any attention. Aren't you lucky!"

Of course, what I mean, quite sincerely is that life is busy and demanding and if you really are "feeling nothing", I am genuinely happy for you. Does it mean you have achieved perfect health? Not at all. For a start, you might be stiff on the other leg, or side.

Second, how is your aerobic fitness, your motor control and your strength? Health, fitness and wellbeing has several components. And, I'm only referring to the physical elements.

What are the other possibilities if you or your student are 'not feeling anything'? First, check that you are performing the material correctly. Next, check that you really are feeling nothing! If you remain still and turn your attention inward for a moment, it's actually pretty hard to feel nothing.

What do you feel, and where do you feel it? Often, this introspection will bring some awareness to the region being stretched, and you might find that indeed there is a stretch happening, albeit a small one.

Related to this is the questions "What are you expecting to feel?" "Do you know what a stretch in this region feels like?" These questions are not meant to deny the truth of self-reports from you or your students. What they are designed to do is encourage a bit more self-enquiry before the stretch is declared ineffective.

And if it is ineffective in the end, so be it. Move onto to a more difficult one, or spend some time on something else entirely. I will not be offended!

What if I can't hold the restretch for 15 breaths?

Students will often claim it is too painful to hold the position for 15 deep breaths. This could be true. So should you give up entirely? No! Just ease out of it a bit. As the teacher of a class, or a self-teacher, try to encourage some self-enquiry during this phase. Ask questions. "How does it feel?", "Where do you feel it?", "Are the sensations continuous, or do they ebb and flow?" "What color are they? Red and hot, or green and comfortable?"

As well as ensuring that the stretches are maximally effective, making students hold the position will, without any doubt, increase their tolerance to pain and discomfort. This in time will improve their stretching outcomes and may carry over into other areas of their lives as well. Indeed, there are numerous MRI brain scans to demonstrate that with repeated exposure to discomfort, so long as your stay with it, your brain will "light up" less and your tolerance will increase.

How do students learn?

Students learn in 3 essential ways: Visually, verbally and kinesthetically (i.e. by feeling and doing). In the beginning of acquiring a skill, the visual and the kinesthetic are by far the most effective. So, don't talk for hours and don't mention anatomical features in Latin! Provide a brief demonstration and let your students explore the material.

Once they are in the stretch, more verbalization will be effective. Freud once said that "we learn through contrast." In this context I believe this to be true.

Allow your students to feel the stretches, and slowly, you can refine them if necessary. They will feel the contrast between stiffness and looseness, tension and relaxation, and 'right and wrong' positioning over time.

You must provide the environment that encourages that kind of kinetic introspection. Be cautious about 'right and wrong' too. If your students feel a stretch, to what extent is it wrong? (See discussions in the books above.)

Which muscles are included & why?

Included is at least one stretch for each muscle group of the body, with variations. The list of muscles included would number hundreds. As you read each stretch, you will see the major muscle groups named and illustrated. The spine is offered in its ranges of movement: flexion, extension, lateral flexion and rotation. We have started at the lower leg, and worked our way up through the body. Of course, you can create your own order.

There are three hamstring stretches. This is to ensure that all of the hip extensors are stretched. Without these three, this would not occur. All up, you have stretches for calves, hamstrings, hip flexors, adductors, glutes, the spine, shoulders & forearms. The muscles of the neck are stretched indirectly in many of the stretches.

Contract/Relax Stretching

Here's how it works:

1 Take yourself VERY SLOWLY into a mild stretch. We call this the POINT OF TENSION, or POT. On a scale of one to ten, one being not much of a stretch and ten being complete agony, we suggest a score of **five or six**. Hold the position for five breaths and settle.
Ask your students to rate the intensity for themselves, if you are teaching a class.

2 Contract the muscles that you are trying to stretch. We will give you cues, of course; although it may seem counterintuitive, contract the muscles we recommend for **five seconds**. Use around 30 % of your maximum effort, and start gently.
Use the cues described freely. If you are teaching and have alternatives, be sure to keep them very simple.

3 Relax totally and restretch to the new position. Don't expect miracles, but you can expect to be able to go further into the stretch, often between 1 to 10 centimetres further. Hold the new POT for **fifteen breaths**.

Here is an example from the posterior stretch:

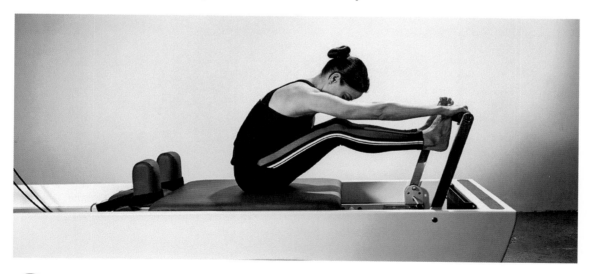

1 Press the carriage away to the POT. Hold for **5 breaths**.

2 Contract the muscles you are stretching. In this case, it is the hamstrings.
Contract for **5 seconds** by pressing your feet down into the foot bar.
Use 30% of maximum force.

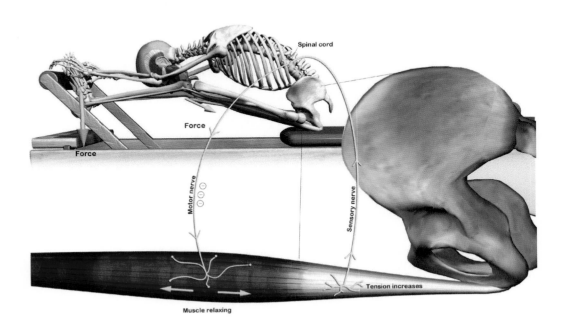

3 Relax and re-stretch to the new POT. Hold for **15 deep breaths**.

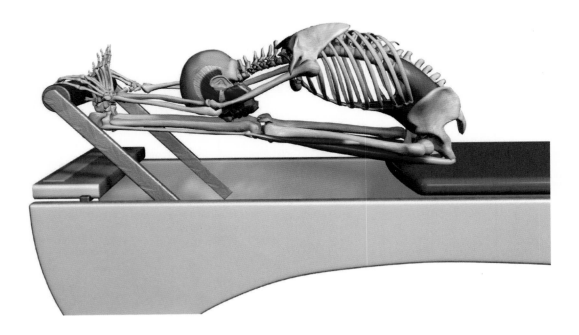

The Calves

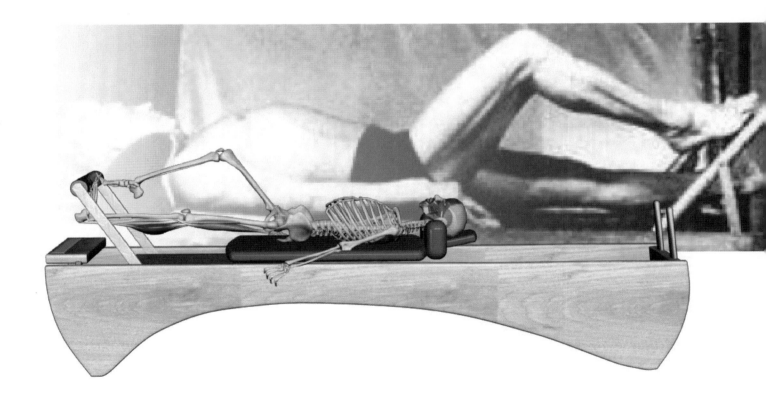

and lower leg compartments

The Lying Calves

- **Standard:** Any • **Spring Tension:** Medium - Heavy
- **Muscle Emphasis:** Entire calf group

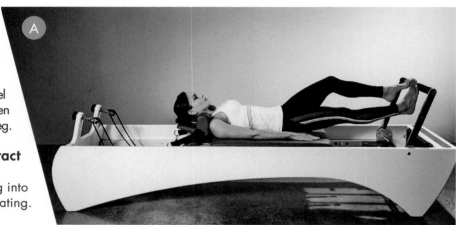

A. How to stretch

Press carriage away and lower one heel slowly to POT. Bend other knee. Tighten quadriceps in stretching leg.

A. How to contract

Press ball of foot that is stretching into foot bar as if accelerating.

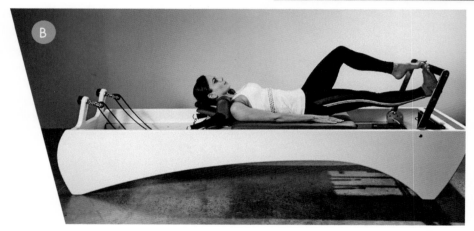

B & C. How to restretch

Lower heel slowly under bar.

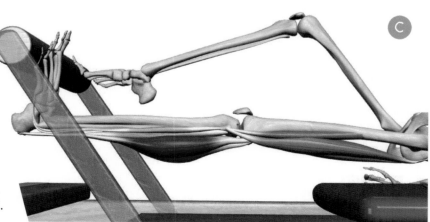

What to watch out for:

- Gripping with toes
- Moving into stretch too quickly -"bouncing".
- Allowing knee to bend.

A partner can intensify this stretch in the gastrocnemius in particular by holding your heel and pulling it gently but firmly under the bar.

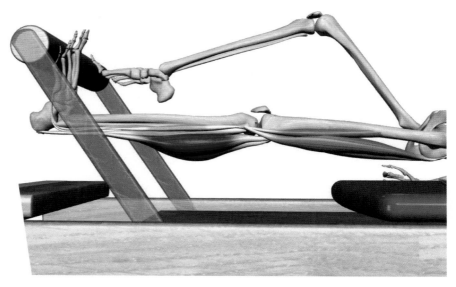

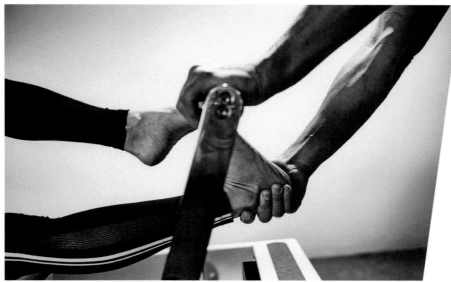

 Please scan QR code to view the video *The Lying Calves*.

Hamstrings

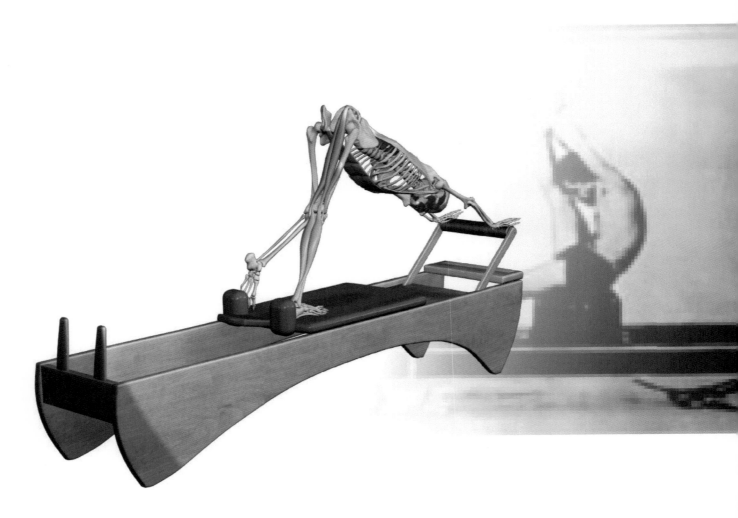

and other hip extensors

Lying HS

- **Standard:** Beginner & Intermediate • **Spring Tension:** Medium
- **Muscle Emphasis:** HS group, gastrocnemius, adductor magnus, horizontal leg-hip flexors

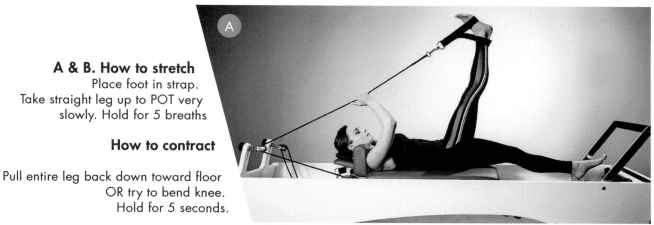

A & B. How to stretch
Place foot in strap.
Take straight leg up to POT very
slowly. Hold for 5 breaths

How to contract
Pull entire leg back down toward floor
OR try to bend knee.
Hold for 5 seconds.

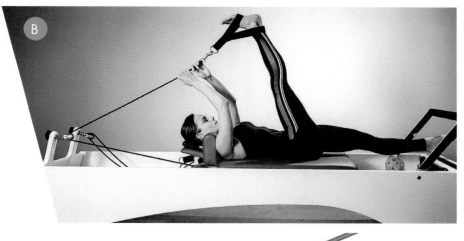

B. How to restretch
On a breath out, allow
carriage to slide in and hip to
flex further.

What to watch out for:
- Legs remain parallel.
- Hips remain square to leg/
neutral pelvis, no posterior or
lateral rotation.
- Legs remain straight.
- Bottom leg remains horizontal.

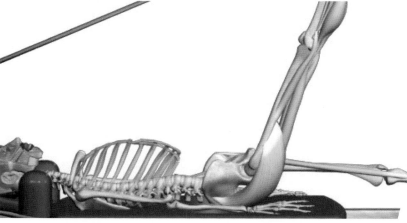

The posterior chain of leg muscles being stretched includes the Gastrocnemius, Hamstrings and extensor fibers of Gluteus Maximus.

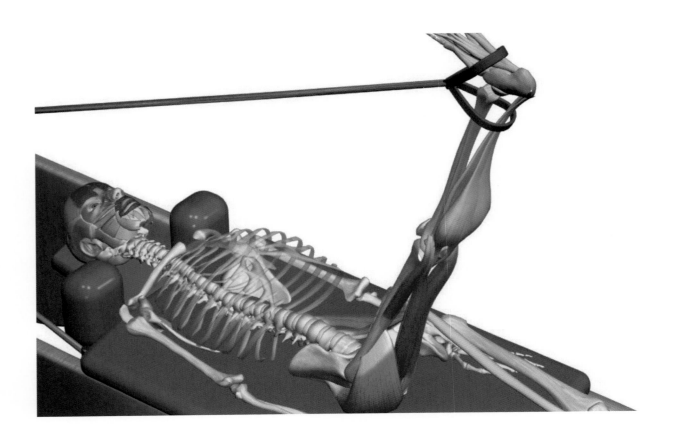

Keep an eye on the horizontal leg too. If it lifts, there could be stifness in sartorious, psoas and others.

Lying Big Toe

- **Standard:** Beginner & Intermediate • **Spring Tension:** Medium
- **Muscle Emphasis:** Bicep femoris both heads, lateral gastrocnemius, external hip rotators, gluteus maximus, medius, minimus, horizontal leg-hip flexors

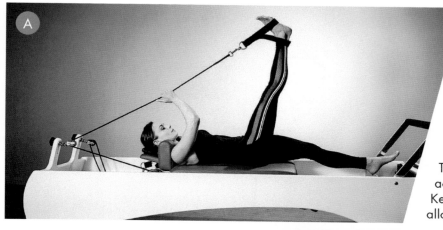

A & B. How to stretch

Take leg into flexion to POT, then slowly across midline of body.
Keep pelvis level horizontally (don't allow hip of lifted leg to lift).

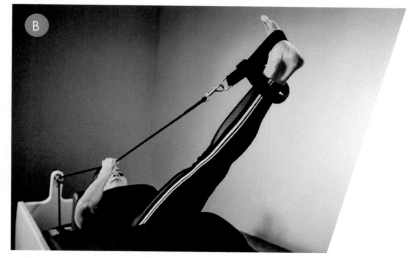

B. How to contract

Press leg diagonally away from stretch position.

C. How to restretch

Take leg further into flexion, and further across midline of body.

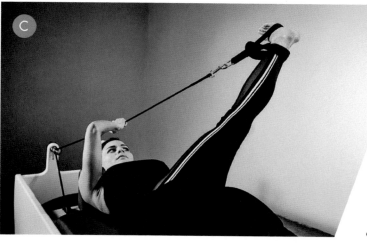

What to watch out for:

- Keep both hips on carriage.
- Keep pelvis neutral.
- Keep bottom leg horizontal.
- Keep stretching leg totally straight.
- Do not allow stretch leg to internally or externally rotate.

The posterior chain of muscles illustrated will stretch. The calves — in particular the lateral head of gastrocnemius, the lateral hamstrings including the short and long head of biceps femoris and even the pirifomis muscle of the hip — may feel a stretch.

The sartorius flexes, abducts and externally rotates the hip joint. If you find your lower leg tending toward any of these positions, stiffness in sartorius may be present.

Similarly, the tensor fascia lata flexes and abducts the thigh. If you show any signs of this motion, make note of it for later inspection.

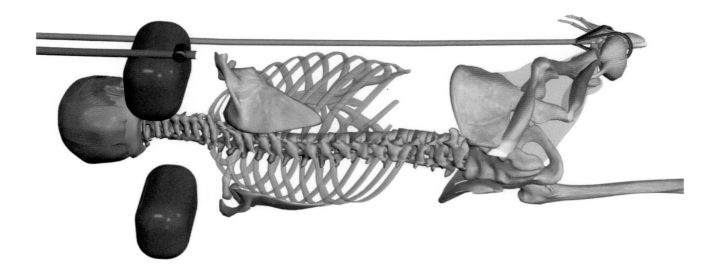

The "worm view" from under the reformer carriage illustrates the piriformis and long head of biceps femoris. You can see that by taking the leg across the body these two muscles will stretch.

Standing HS Bent Leg

- **Standard:** Beginner & Intermediate • **Spring Tension:** Light to Medium
- **Muscle Emphasis:** HS group, gluteus maximus-extensor fibers, adductor magnus, rear leg hip flexors

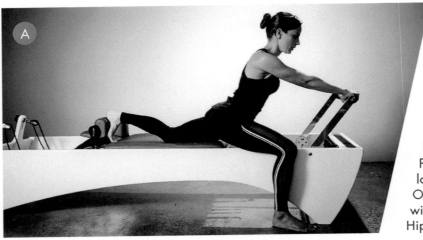

A & B. How to stretch

Place foot on floor toward front of reformer. Press carriage away with rear leg and lower hips maximally with front knee bent. Once in position, try to straighten front leg without lifting hips to POT.
Hips must remain square to line of rear leg.

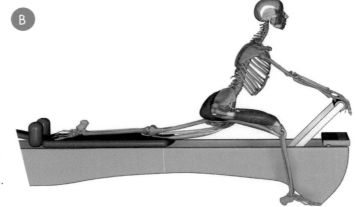

B. How to contract

Press both feet down.

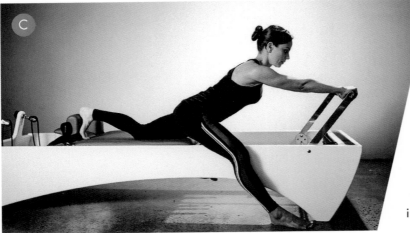

C. How to restretch

Slide carriage further out by trying to straighten front leg. Place hands either on bar or side of reformer.

What to watch out for:

- Hips lifting.
- Not lowering hips maximally in initial position.

Use This Link to See Video: https://www.youtube.com/watch?v=-mIVVwA4vlc

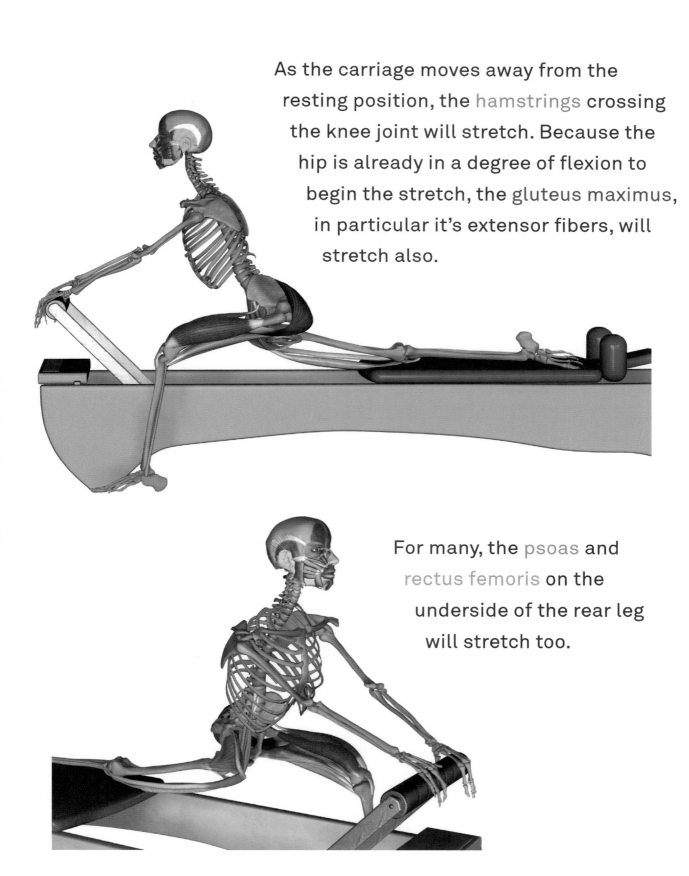

As the carriage moves away from the resting position, the hamstrings crossing the knee joint will stretch. Because the hip is already in a degree of flexion to begin the stretch, the gluteus maximus, in particular it's extensor fibers, will stretch also.

For many, the psoas and rectus femoris on the underside of the rear leg will stretch too.

Hip Flexors

& Quadriceps

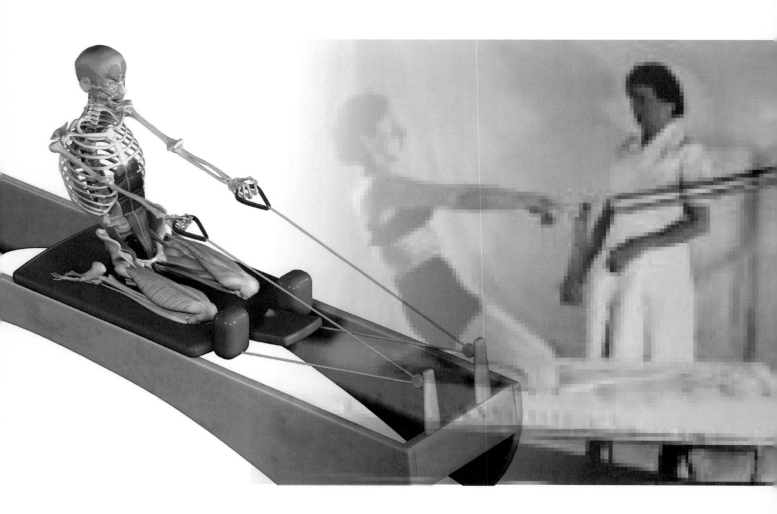

The Standing Lunge

- **Standard:** Beginner • **Spring Tension:** Light-Medium
- **Muscle Emphasis:** Illiopsoas, rectus femoris, secondary-underside of front leg-hamstrings, gluteus maximus, adductor magnus

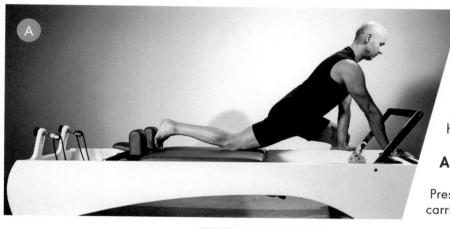

A. How to stretch

Press carriage away, bend front knee and lower hips maximally. Use arms to support body weight. Ensure hips stay square to line of legs.

A. How to contract

Press back foot and knee down into carriage, and front foot.

B & C. How to restretch

Lower hips further. Tilt pelvis toward posterior tilt. Lift rear knee without lifting hips (Photo C). Contract abdominals.

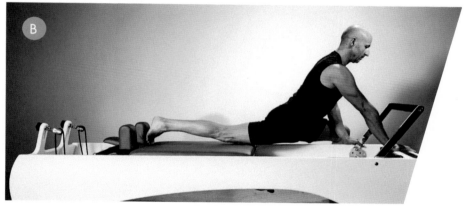

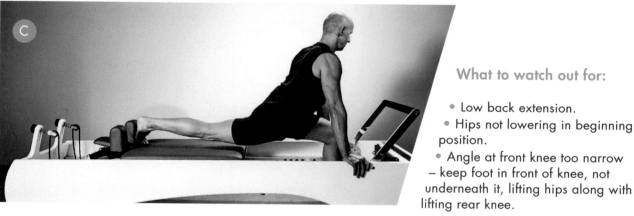

What to watch out for:

- Low back extension.
- Hips not lowering in beginning position.
- Angle at front knee too narrow – keep foot in front of knee, not underneath it, lifting hips along with lifting rear knee.

◀ Please scan QR code to view the video *The Standing Lunge.*

The Lunge 3.0 with Rec Fem & Quads

- **Standard:** Intermediate to Advanced • **Spring Tension:** Light - Medium
- **Muscle Emphasis:** Illiopsoas, rectus femoris, quadriceps, secondary- underside of front leg-hamstrings, gluteus maximus, adductor magnus

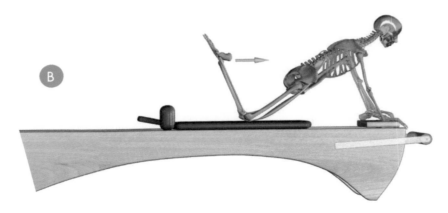

A. How to stretch

Press carriage away, bend front knee to just over 90 degrees. Lower hips maximally. Press back leg away while maintaining angle at front leg.

Place hands inside front leg. Lift back foot slowly toward bottom. Partner to press on pelvis to keep hips low.

B. How to contract

Press back foot away from bottom. Press back knee down into carriage. Press front foot into reformer.

C. How to restretch

Lower hips further.
Take rear foot toward bottom.

What to watch out for:

- Hips not lowering in beginning position.
- Angle at front knee too narrow.
- Leaning hips backward.

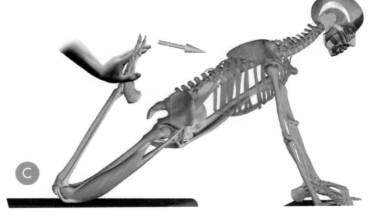

 ◀ Please scan QR code to view the video *The Standing Lunge 3.0.*

Gluteals

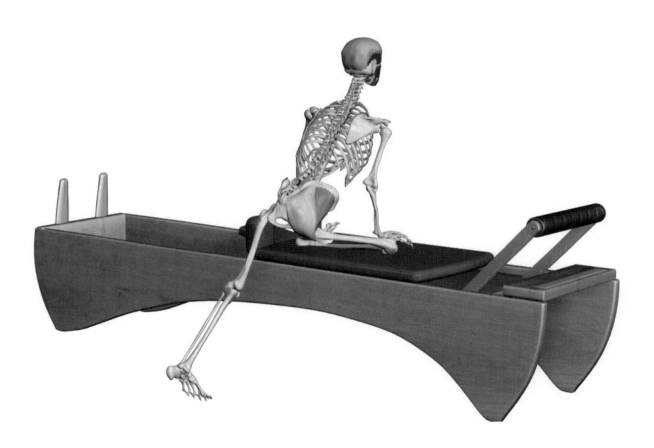

The Lying Gluteals

- **Standard:** Beginner • **Spring Tension:** Medium
- **Muscle Emphasis:** Gluteal group including deep hip rotators

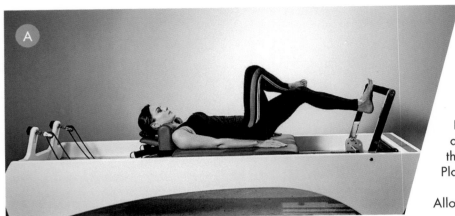

A & B. How to stretch

Press carriage away, bend knee and place ankle onto opposite thigh. Pelvis must remain neutral. Place hand under low back to assist.

Allow carriage to return to POT.

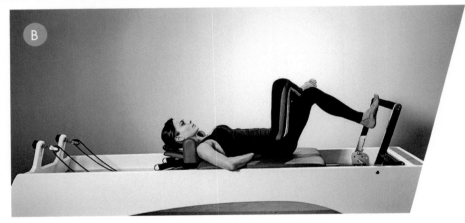

B. How to contract

Press ankle into thigh.

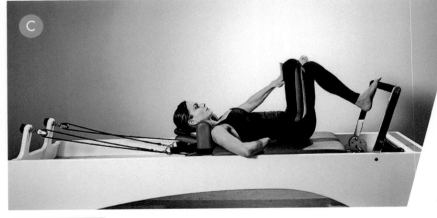

C. How to restretch

Allow carriage to move further toward foot bar.
Press knee of stretching leg away.

What to watch out for:

- Low back flattening.
- Bottom lifting/posterior pelvic rotation.
- Lateral pelvic rotation.

◀ Please scan QR code to view the video *The Lying Gluteals*.

Adductors

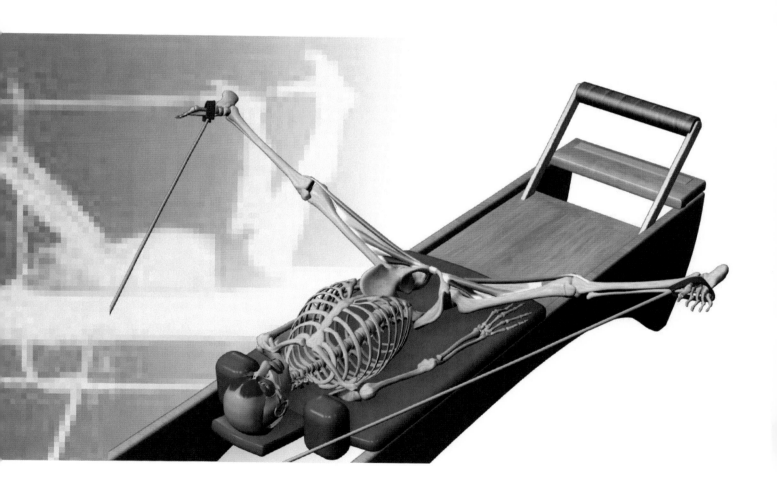

The Lying Splits

- **Standard:** Any • **Spring Tension:** Medium
- **Muscle Emphasis:** Entire adductor group and medial hamstrings

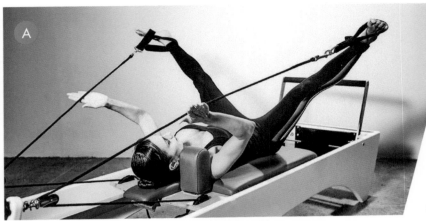

A. How to stretch

Take legs to 90 degrees from floor. Hold straps to enable legs to slowly come apart to POT.

Release straps from hands if comfortable (not shown).

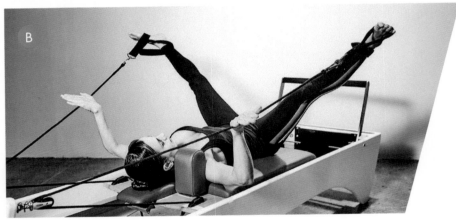

B. How to contract

Press legs back together and prevent any movement with hands.

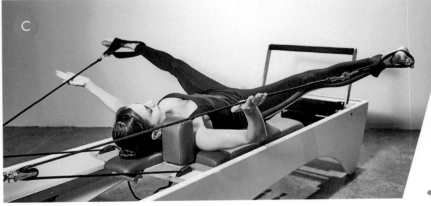

C. How to restretch

Allow legs to fall further apart. Use arms to press down onto straps for greater effect.

What to watch out for:

- Legs not at 90 degrees to begin.
- Not allowing legs to relax.
- Moving into stretch too quickly.

◀ Please scan QR code to view the video *The Lying Splits.*

As the leg moves into more flexion (i.e. the feet moving toward the back end of the reformer), the posterior adductors like adductor magnus are stretched more strongly. Gracilis is the longest adductor, acting on both the knee and hip joints.

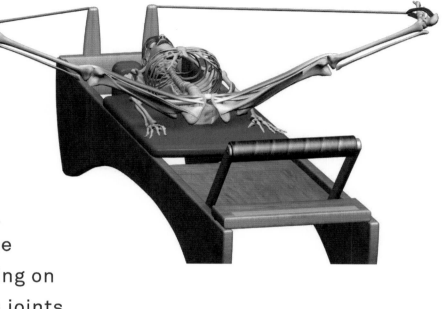

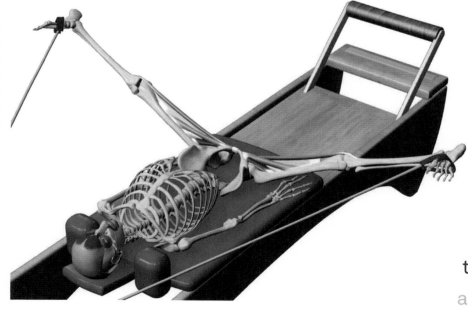

Topographically, the adductor muscles are organised into three layers. The most superficial layer can be seen here and includes the pectineus, adductor longus and gracilis.

Variations to Effect Different Adductors

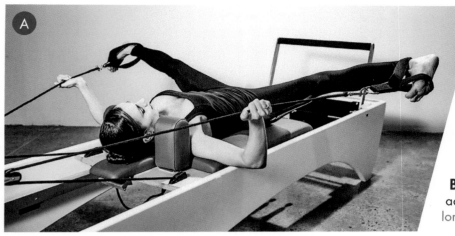

A. Externally rotate the legs for posterior adductors: adductor magnus.

B. Internally rotate legs for anterior adductors: pectineus and adductor longus.

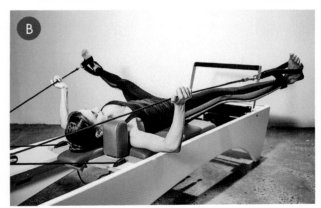

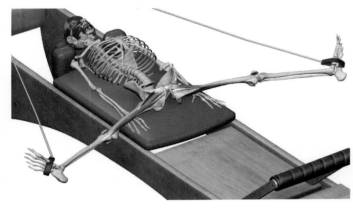

Variation Two

For muscle imbalances, bend one knee and allow the stretch to be felt mostly in the straight leg.

Straight leg can be taken into more or fewer degrees of hip flexion depending on sensations and requirements.

Greater hip flexion will translate to more effects on hamstrings and posterior adductors. See images above.

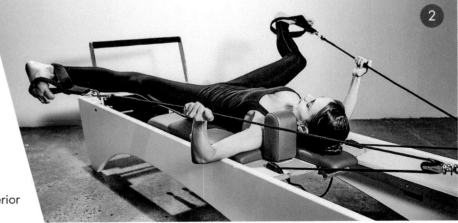

The Spine

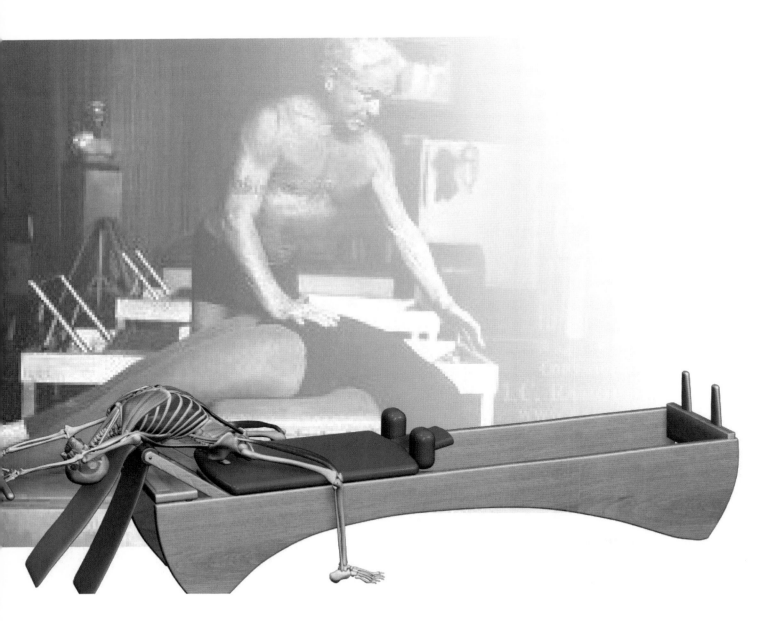

The Posterior Stretch

- **Standard:** Beginner • **Spring Tension:** Light - Medium
- **Muscle Emphasis:** All spinal extensors from superficial to deep, hamstrings, calves, adductor magnus, gluteus maximus, latissimus dorsi

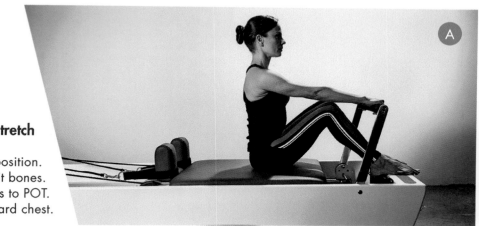

A & B. How to stretch

Sit with feet on lower position.
Align feet with sit bones.
Slowly try to straighten legs to POT.
Take chin toward chest.

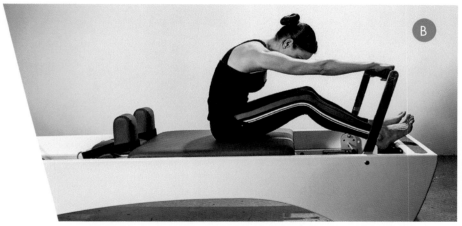

B. How to contract

Press feet down into reformer.

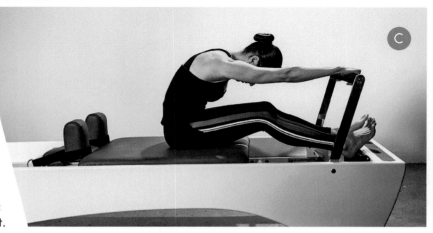

C. How to restretch

Straighten legs further.

What to watch out for:

- Moving carriage out too fast.
  - Not taking chin to chest.
  - Too much flexion in thoracic spine and legs still bent.

As you straighten your legs, the entire chain of muscles on the posterior surface of your body will stretch.

The calf group, the hamstrings and the entire erector spinae group will stretch. Because of the fascial interconnectedness of these groups, tension in one area can be transmitted to another region.

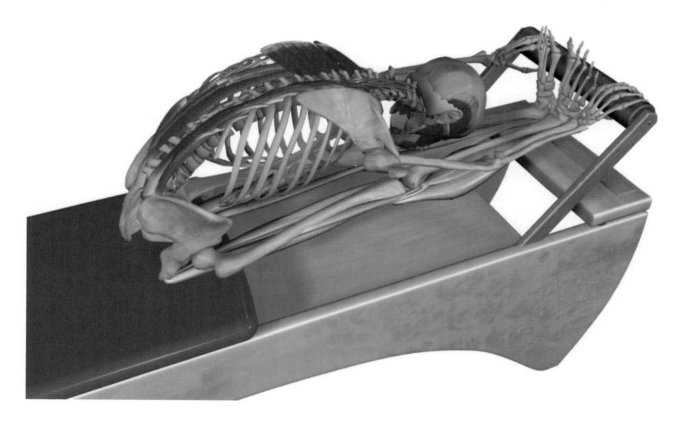

Note for teachers: Common postural compensation patterns associated with tightness in this posterior chain include ankle dorsiflexion restriction, knee hyperextension, hamstring shortness, sacral nutation, upper cervical hyperextension and rotation of the occiput.

The latissimus dorsi, a large and important muscle on the back and arms, will often be stretched here too.

In conjunction with the transverses abdominus, the latissimus can be used to safeguard your spine if you feel it is vulnerable during this stretch.

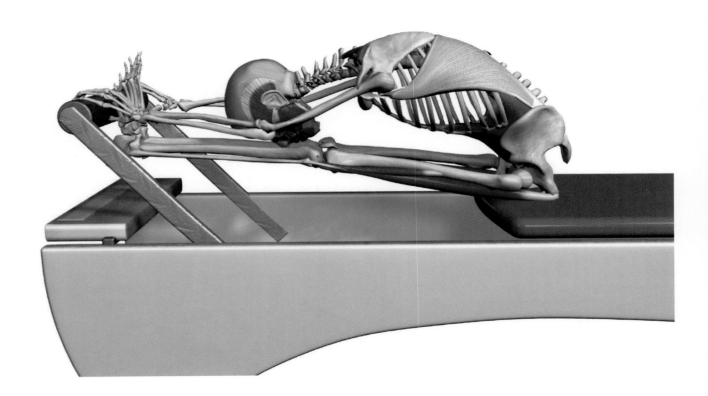

Please take our "Safeguarding the Spine" online workshop for tips and cues on integrating a greater strength element into this stretch.

 "Safeguarding the Spine" Workshop at www.innovationsinpilates.com

Because a portion of the large and powerful gluteus maximus attach onto the leg bone or femur, they will be stretched in this position also.

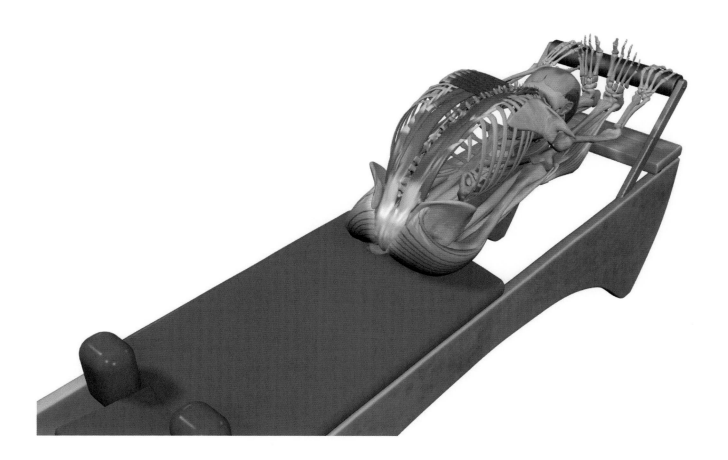

If you are tight, and your shoulder blades rotate upwardly, your rhomboids will also feel a degree of stretch.

The Pull Push

- Standard: Any • Spring Tension: No Springs
- Muscle Emphasis: All spinal extensors, rhomboids, middle & upper trapezius, levato scapular

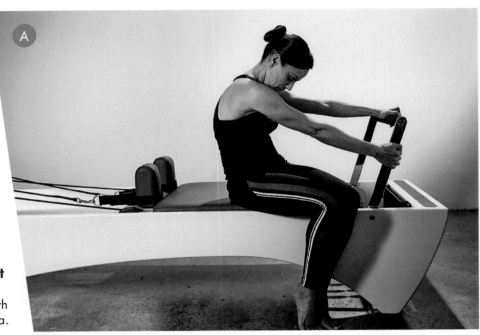

A. How to stretch

Sit on oblique angle to foot bar. Roll pelvis backward/ posteriorly strongly to ensure carriage does not move by sending pubic bone toward foot bar. Place hands on bar as pictured. Pull lightly with arm on sidebar. Push strongly with arm into foot bar. Take chin toward chest. Lean whole body backwards strongly.

A. How to contract

Pull on sidebar with arm trying to retract scapula.

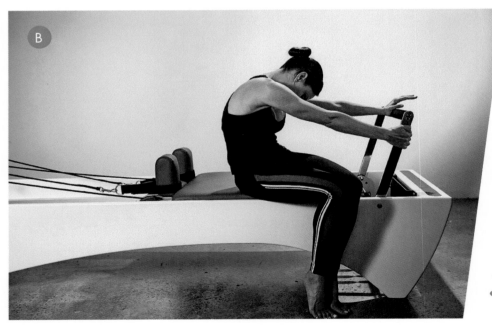

B. How to restretch
Lean back further. Tighten abdominal muscles. Tilt ear toward top (left in photo) arm.

What to watch out for:

- Carriage moving out.
- Not taking chin to chest.
- Not leaning backwards.
- Not thrusting pelvis toward footbar.

Please scan QR code to view the video *The Pull Push.*

The middle and upper trapezius muscles will stretch, along with the rhomboids; mostly on the side with the arm on the side bar. Be sure to swap and do both sides.

As you take your chin toward your chest, your levator scapula and splenius capitis muscles will also be stretched.

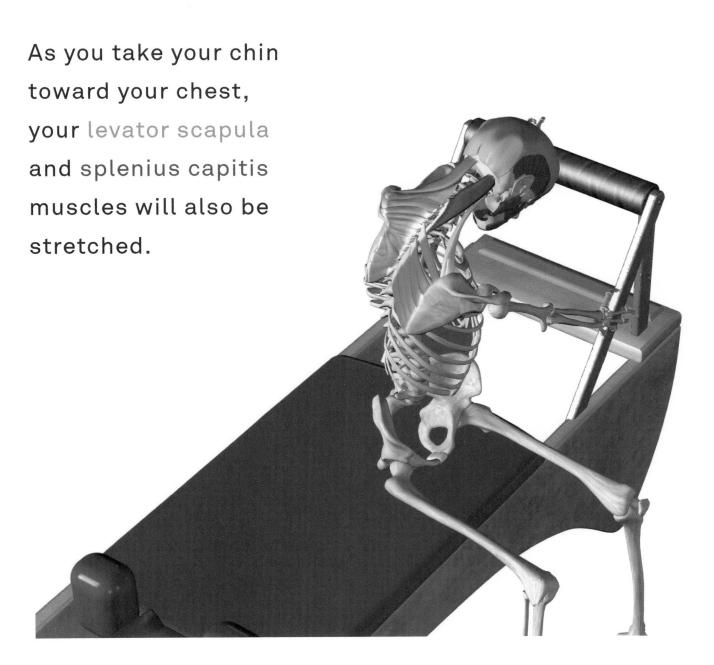

Lying Rotation

- **Standard:** Any • **Spring Tension:** Heavy
- **Muscle Emphasis:** Pectorals, anterior deltoid, serratus anterior, spinal extensors, oblique abdominals, gluteal group, abductors

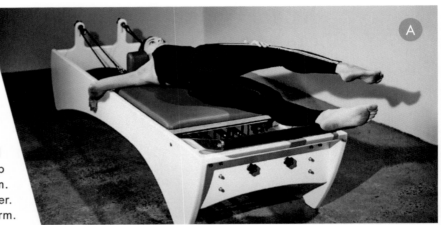

A. How to stretch

Hook hand under or onto side of reformer and lower the elbow. Move opposite hip bone to centre of carriage to maintain spinal alignment/elongation. Rotate hip and leg away from top arm. Drape leg over side of reformer. Press down on leg with free arm.

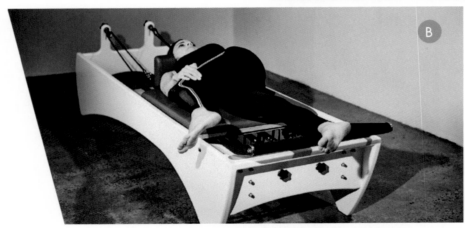

B. How to contract

Press arm up into reformer. Press top leg back into free arm.

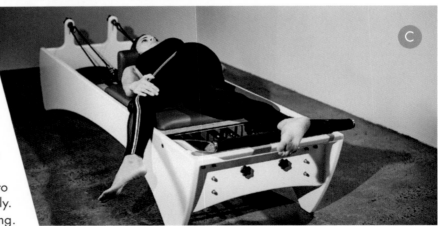

C. How to restretch

Twist further into rotated position. Press bent knee down.

What to watch out for:

- Not shifting hip to center of carriage initially.
- Shallow breathing.

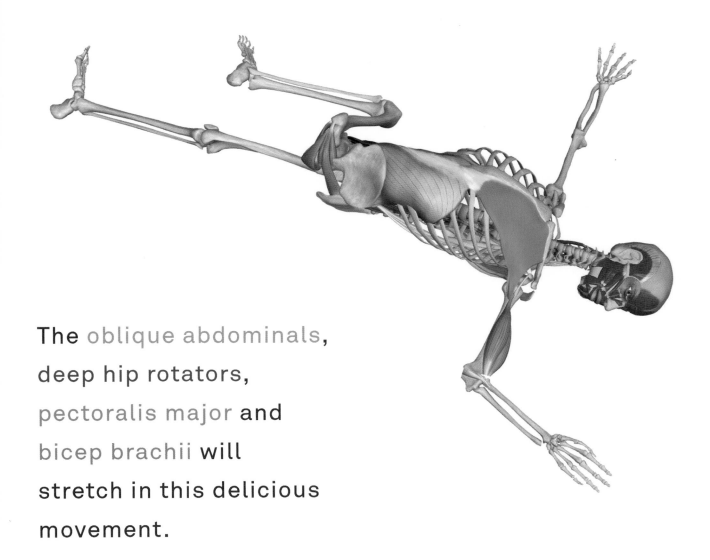

The oblique abdominals, deep hip rotators, pectoralis major and bicep brachii will stretch in this delicious movement.

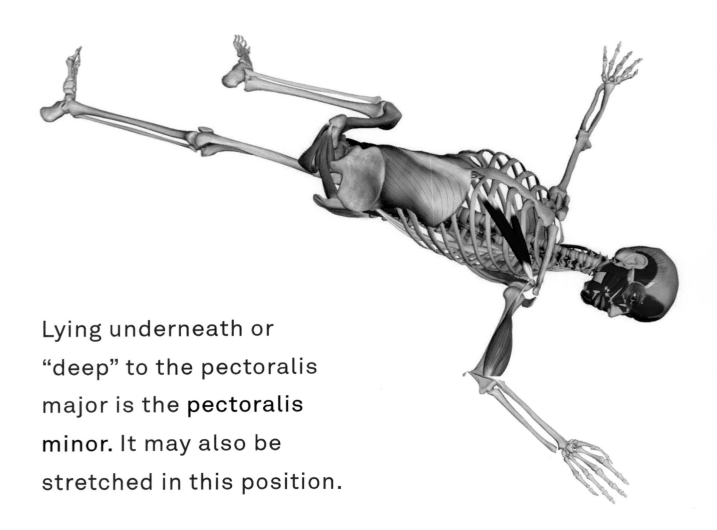

Lying underneath or "deep" to the pectoralis major is the **pectoralis minor**. It may also be stretched in this position.

The Mermaid

- **Standard:** Beginner/Intermediate • **Spring Tension:** Light - Medium
- **Muscle Emphasis:** Oblique abdominals, quadratus lumborum, intercostals, abductors

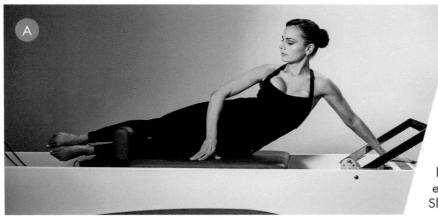

A & B. How to stretch

Slide carriage out and sit in center.
Place top leg/foot on top of bottom
leg/foot. Align feet, hips, hand,
ensure top hip above bottom hip.
Slide carriage in to POT to find stretch.

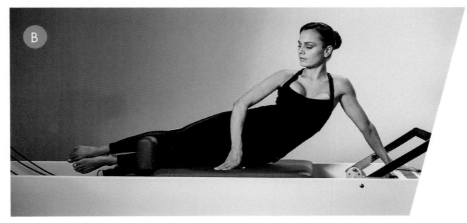

B. How to contract

Press hands and feet
down into floor.

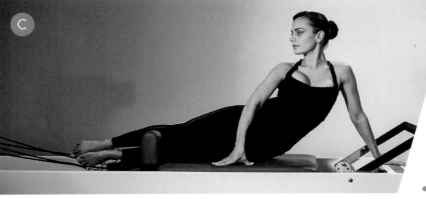

C. How to restretch

Slide carriage in further.
Deepen inhalations as
much as possible.

What to watch out for:

- Not aligning top hip with feet.

◀ Please scan QR code to view the video *The Mermaid.*

Variations

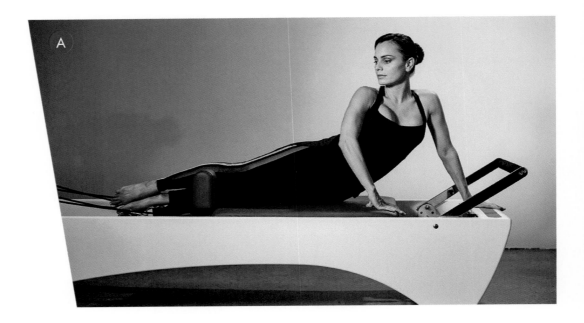

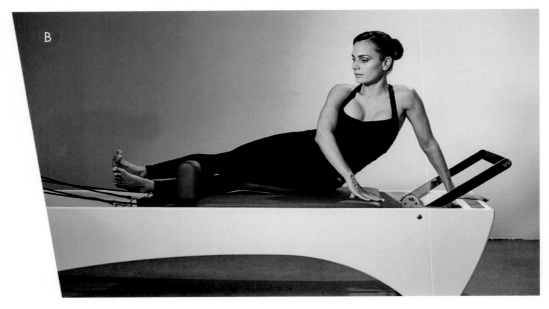

Roll top hip forward (A) and backward (B)
to shift stretch around.

As the carriage slides in, the spine is bent further sideways. The internal obliques will stretch along with the hip abductors gluteus medius and minimus, the quadatus lumborum and half of the erector spinae group.

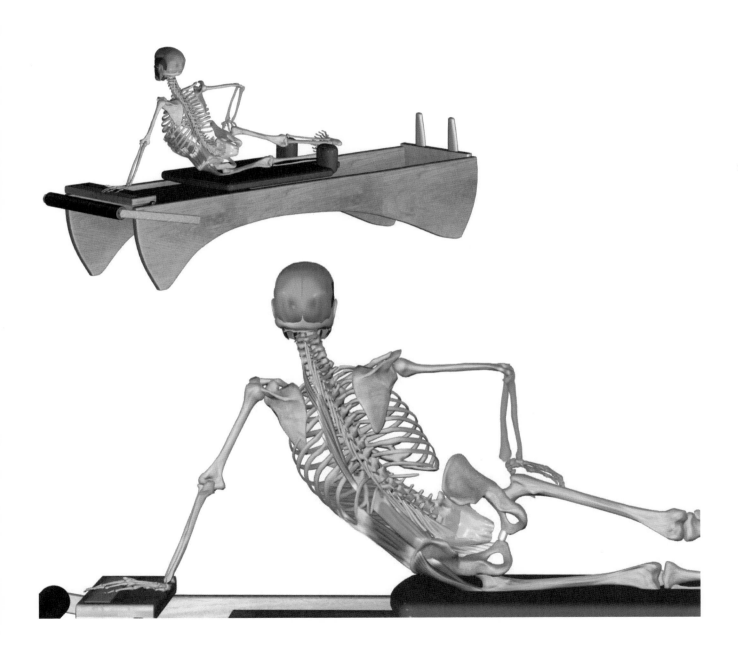

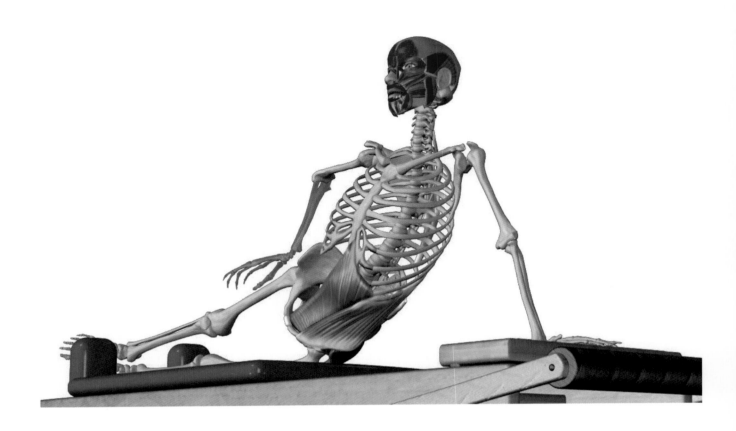

The internal obliques, lying "deep" to or underneath the external obliques, will also be stretched as you explore different hip angles.

Deep inhalations will increase the stretch. As the diaphragm descends, it will push the non-compressible abdominal content out towards the obliques, stretching them further.

Seated Backbend

- **Standard:** Beginner/Intermediate • **Spring Tension:** Heavy
- **Muscle Emphasis:** Psoas, rectus femoris, abdominals, pectorals, lats, anterior neck, triceps long head, rotator cuff

How to stretch

Place secure box close to foot bar to support head.
Sit on carriage close to footbar.
Sit back so that bar is just below scapula/shoulder blades.
Take hands and head back slowly.

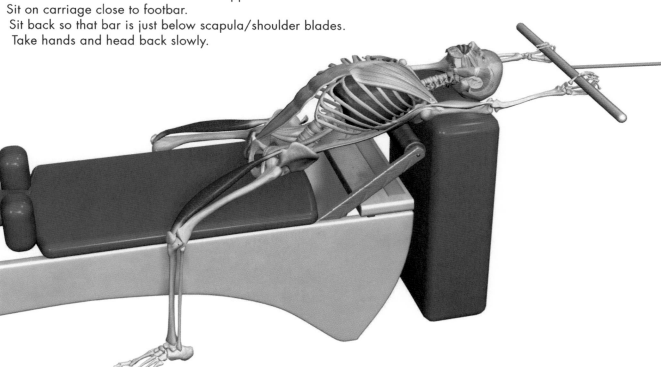

How to contract

Press hands and thighs up toward ceiling.

How to restretch

Allow pelvis, legs and arms to drop/flop.
Partner can pull arms downward and alternately pull one side more.

What to watch out for:

- Unnecessary tension in arms, neck, stomach.
- Dizziness is a strong sign to stop immediately.

◀ Please scan QR code to view the video *The Seated Backbend.*

Arms & Shoulders

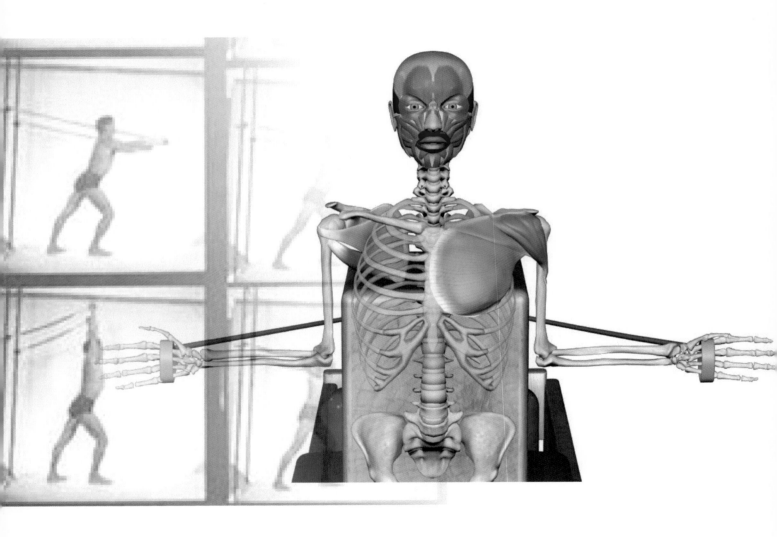

The Wrist Flexors

- **Standard:** Any • **Spring Tension:** no springs
- **Muscle Emphasis:** All wrist flexors

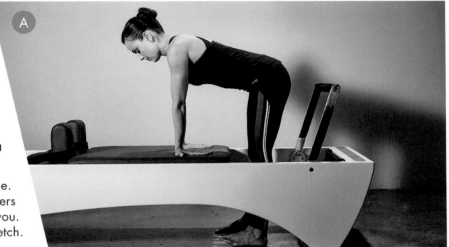

A. How to stretch

Stand inside reformer frame.
Place palms onto carriage with fingers
facing toward you.
Slide carriage out to find stretch.

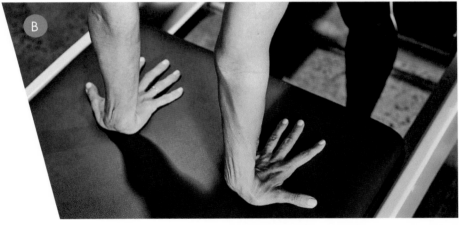

A & B. How to contract

Press palms and fingers down
into carriage.

C. How to restretch

Slide carraige away further.

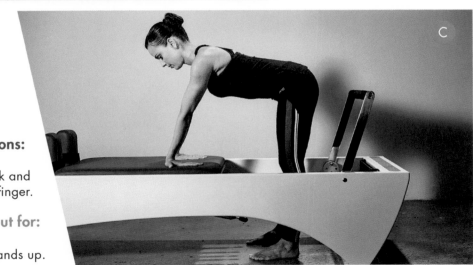

Variations:

Shift weight back and
around above each finger.

What to watch out for:

- Lifting palms of hands up.

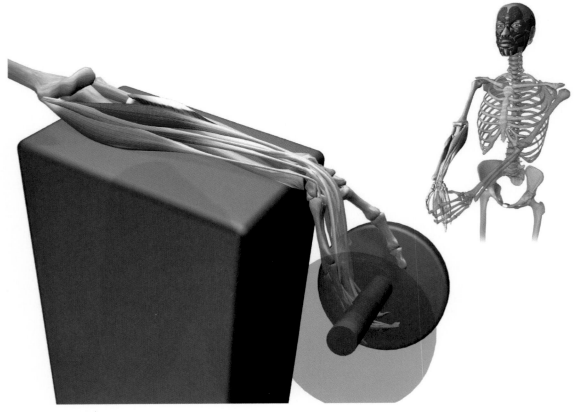

The forearm has both primary and secondary muscles that flex the wrist. You can see some of them attaching just above the inside of the elbow, or medial epicondyle, and running across the wrist as they become tendinous. This region is known as the carpal tunnel, where nine flexor tendons pass though this small compartment. Stretching will help to prevent carpel tunnel syndrome.

The Wrist Extensors

- **Standard:** Any • **Spring Tension:** no springs
- **Muscle Emphasis:** All wrist extensors

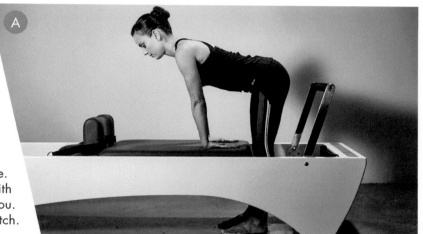

A. How to stretch

Stand inside reformer frame.
Place back of hands onto carriage with
fingers facing toward you.
Slide carriage out to find stretch.

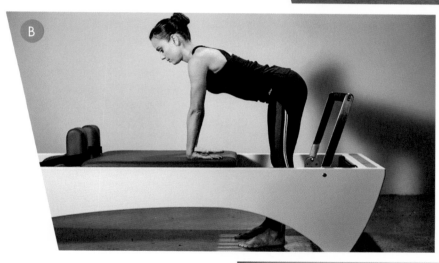

B. How to contract

Press back of hands and
fingers down into carriage.

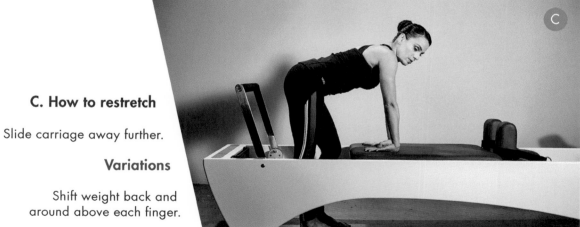

C. How to restretch

Slide carriage away further.

Variations

Shift weight back and
around above each finger.

Internal Shoulder Rotators

- **Standard:** Any • **Spring Tension:** Medium to Heavy
- **Muscle Emphasis:** Teres major, subscapularis, anterior deltoid, clavicular portion of pectoralis major

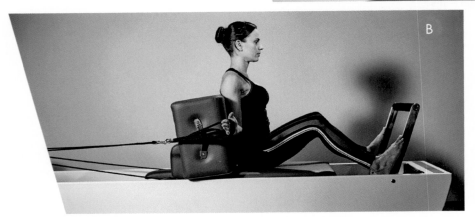

A. How to stretch

Sit on carriage in front of box.
Bend elbows to 90 degrees.
Keep upper arms close to body.
Allow carriage to slide in to
find stretch in shoulders.
Use feet to control carriage movement.

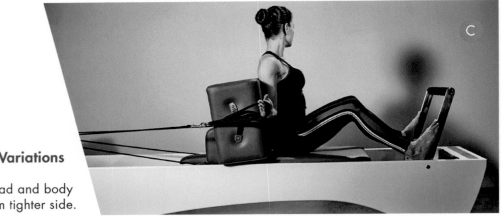

A. How to contract

Press hands into straps in
clapping motion.

B. How to restretch

Slide carriage further in.
Control movement with legs.

C. Variations

Carefully turn head and body
away from tighter side.

 Please scan QR code to view the video *Internal Shoulder Rotators.*

No Box?

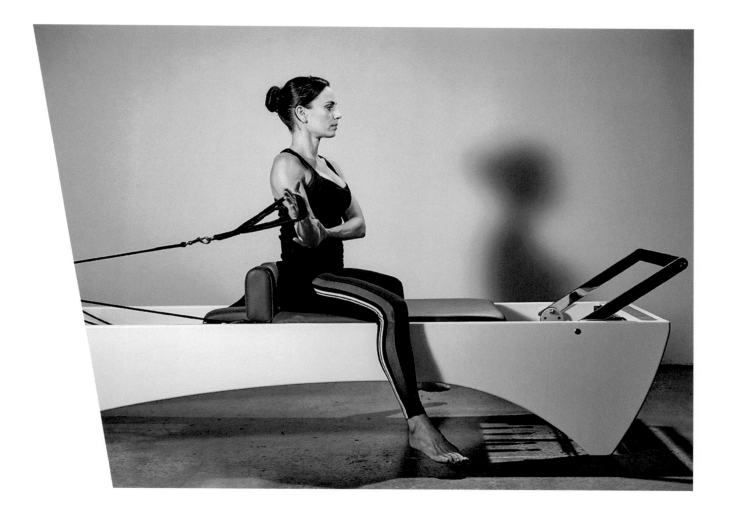

Reach around and hold your elbow with one hand and keep it from moving. Allow the carriage to slide in as above.

The subscapularis and teres major are the two muscles stretched the most. The sensations may not be precise, but will stem from anywhere round the shoulder joint.

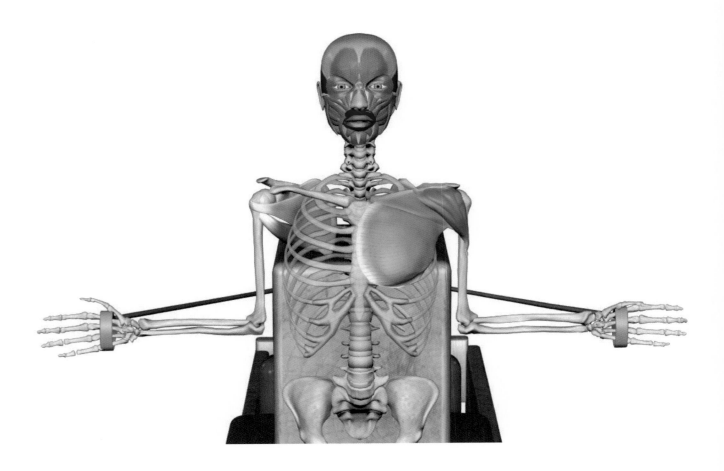

If you are tight, the pectoralis major – in particular its costal fibers – may stretch, as well as the anterior deltoid.

Conclusion

Some other suggestions about using this material

"If you can't explain it simply, you don't understand it well enough."
Einstein

There is easily enough material here for a 60 to 90 minute Innovations in Pilates class. There is months, if not years of practice to be able to teach the material with ease as well. I have always believed that you should 'own' an exercise before you teach it. That is, you should have a pretty accomplished practice including the awareness of how it feels before you consider teaching it to others. You should also have the practiced cuing vocabulary to make the exercise accessible to others.

In this respect, I have quoted Einstein before: "If you can't explain it simply, you don't understand it well enough." It is a truism that the more you know an exercise, in every dimension of "knowing" (in a feeling sense, a biomechanical sense and a descriptive sense) the better and more simply you can teach it. Bottom line: practice teaching and performing

the material. As you perform it, teach yourself as if you were teaching someone else to develop the vocabulary.

If you are teaching Pilates, feel free to cut and paste this material into your sessions. What I mean by that is that after you have performed some calf work for example, throw in the lying calf stretch. Likewise, do the same for any part of the body. If you have just performed 'chest expansion' for example, try the pull/push for your rhomboids and mid-trapezius muscles.

True body health is a balance of strength and flexibility among other things, so devote time to both. Many in today's world have enough strength to perform the activities of daily life, (as diminished as they may be) but increasingly lack the range of movement to perform them. So an unfortunate, but preventable downward spiral of less movement and atrophied muscle and bone mass, with increased body fat, is perpetuated.

Finally, the principle that has always guided my prescription of exercise is known as the **S.A.I.D principle**. It stands for the Specific Adaptation to Imposed Demands. What it means, and what any enquiry into the mind and body are increasingly demonstrating is that whatever stress we expose ourselves to, we adapt in highly specific ways.

If we perform arm curls at a specific joint angle for example, we become stronger at that joint angle only. If we take up long distance running, we do not improve at sprinting. In fact, we may get slower. If we memorize maps like taxi drivers do, the region of our brains that records such information becomes enlarged.

Interestingly though, taxi drivers only become better at spacial and geographical tasks. Their memory for language for instance, is not increased. So, our adaptations are highly specific.

Think this through before you practice any exercise. Ask yourself this fundamental question "What kind of adaptation am I trying to bring about with this exercise?" If it is what you think you need, go ahead! If it is not, it's time for a re-think.

Enjoy the material and the practice. Keep in touch online for updates, videos, workshops and articles. Better still, join us at a workshop or retreat, practice with us in person, and learn all of our material!

As always, stay loose!

Anthony & Kenyi

Thank You!

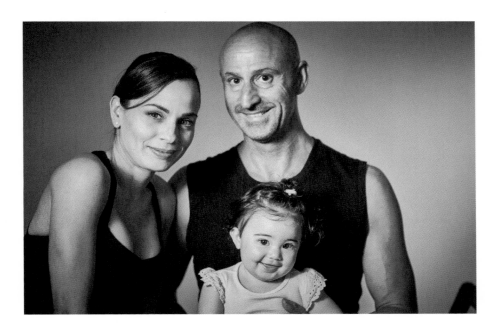

Dear Readers,

Thank you for reading a practicing our material.

Please keep in touch via email: anthony@innovationsinpilates.com
or Facebook: https://www.facebook.com/anthony.lett1
and https://www.facebook.com/Innovations-in-Pilates-519771898058940/

Website: www.innovationsinpilates.com

We have lots of materials: videos, online workshops, books, certifications and retreats.

As always, stay loose!

Warm regards from Anthony, Kenyi and Grace.

Printed in Great Britain
by Amazon